Witches, Midwives & Nurses

BARBARA EHRENREICH
& DEIRDRE ENGLISH

Witches, Midwives & Nurses

A History of Women Healers

SECOND EDITION

FEMINIST PRESS
AT THE CITY UNIVERSITY OF NEW YORK
FEMINISTPRESS.ORG

Published in 2010 by the Feminist Press
at the City University of New York
The Graduate Center
365 Fifth Avenue, Suite 5406
New York, NY 10016

feministpress.org

First Feminist Press edition published 1973
Second edition with new introduction published July 2010
Ninth printing, September 2023

Cover design by John Yates/Stealworks
Text design by Drew Stevens

Library of Congress Cataloging-in-Publication Data

Ehrenreich, Barbara.
 Witches, midwives, and nurses : a history of women healers / Barbara
Ehrenreich and Deirdre English. -- 2nd ed.
   p. ; cm.
 ISBN 978-1-55861-661-5
1. Women in medicine--History. 2. Medicine--United States--History. 3. Women
healers--United States--History. I. English, Deirdre. II. Title.
 [DNLM: 1. History of Nursing--United States. 2. Nurses--United States.
3. Midwifery--history--United States. 4. Witchcraft--history--United States.
5. Women's Health--history--United States. WQ 11 AA1 E33w 2010]
 R692.E35 2010
 610.82--dc22

                                                        2010009446

Contents

Introduction to the Second Edition: The Backstory

WITCHES, MIDWIVES & NURSES (*WMN*) IS A DOCUMENT from the second wave of feminism in the United States. Rereading it forty years later, we find it startling in its assertiveness and sweep and, for the most part, surprisingly accurate, given the paucity of materials we originally had to work with. At the same time, we also cringe a little at what read now like overstatements and overly militant ways of stating things. A lot has changed in forty years, both historically and in our approach to scholarship, so we have to remind ourselves that *WMN* was written in a blaze of anger and indignation. If some of the sources of our anger now seem quaint, this is only because of works like *WMN* and the movement it came out of.

By the early 1970s feminists were becoming aware of a variety of ways women were abused or treated unjustly by the medical system. As health care professionals, women were largely confined to subordinate roles as nurses and aides. As consumers of care, we found ourselves subject to both insensitive and hazardous treatment: unnecessary hysterectomies, over-medicated childbirth, insufficiently tested contraceptives, involuntary sterilizations, and the almost universal condescension of male doctors.

We were not supposed to know anything about our own bodies or to participate in decision-making about our own care. As girls, the women of our generation had grown up thinking of their reproductive organs as the unmentionable region "down there." In the *Ladies' Home Journal*, which many of our mothers read, the medical advice column was entitled "Tell Me, Doctor." Women who asked too many questions or insisted, for example, on "natural" childbirth, frequently found themselves labeled, right in their medical records, as uncooperative or neurotic. Serious complaints were likely to be dismissed as "psychosomatic" and attributed to women's assumed suggestibility. In the standard surgical protocol for breast cancer treatment, the patient was biopsied and then, if the result was positive, rushed into a radical mastectomy without ever being wakened from anesthesia to discuss her options.

One of our first projects in the emerging "women's health movement" was to confront women's ignorance of their own bodies. In Boston, a group of feminists had launched a series of "Know Your Body" courses aimed at the general public—the core of which became the groundbreaking book *Our Bodies, Ourselves* in 1970—and we helped put together a similar course in New York City. A small group of us got together and studied medical textbooks to prepare presentations on such topics as the menstrual cycle, pregnancy, and menopause. Today of course, anyone can learn about these things in high school courses, by reading women's magazines, or just by googling. But at the time, women packed our evening classes, eager for whatever information we had to offer.

We were beginning to suspect that women had not always, in all circumstances, been so disempowered with respect to their own bodies and care. After all, medical technology and the medical profession that monopolized it were relatively recent historical developments, and yet somehow our female ancestors had, however imperfectly, negotiated the challenges of the female life cycle. Having met as teachers at a new branch of the State University of New York, the College at Old Westbury—which was devoted at the time to "nontraditional" students, usually in their twenties or older, for the most part black and Hispanic—we had an opportunity to satisfy our curiosity. The campus was then a hotbed of political debate over class, race, gender, and "identity politics," with Florence Howe, who went on to launch the Feminist Press, working to develop what was one of the first women's studies programs in the nation. Encouraged by her and other colleagues, we created a course on women's health, which gave us an excuse to read up on the history of women and medicine.

There was not a lot to read at the time, the entire genre of books on "Women and . . ." having yet to be invented. Sometimes, in conventional histories of American medicine, we found tantalizing references to a time when women predominated as healers—but only as an indication of how "primitive" American medicine had been before the rise of the modern medical profession. What kept us going was the powerful reinforcement we were getting from our students, many of them practical nurses seeking RN degrees, who often brought with them memories and experiences of female healing traditions: we had midwives from the Caribbean, baffled by the then near nonexistence of midwifery in this country, women from European immigrant backgrounds who could recall grandmothers who practiced lay healing arts, and African Americans who carried memories of an autonomous black midwifery tradition in the American south.

Sometime in 1972—and we are both hazy on exactly when—we were invited to attend a small conference on women's health held in rural Pennsylvania. This, it seemed, was our chance to test our emerging hypotheses on an audience of activists and a few fledgling scholars. We no longer possess the mimeographed outline of our findings that we took to the conference, but the central idea was that the medical profession as we knew it (still over 90 percent male) had replaced and driven out a much older tradition of female lay healing, including both midwifery and a range of healing skills, while closing medical education to women. In other words, the ignorance and disempowerment of women that we confronted in the 1970s were not longstanding conditions, but were the result of a prolonged power struggle that had taken place in America in the early nineteenth century, well before the rise of scientific medicine. We traced a similar power struggle in Europe back to the early modern era and, inspired in part by the wonderfully iconoclastic Thomas Szasz, we looked at how female lay healers of the same era were frequently targeted as "witches."

The response to our presentation was sufficiently enthusiastic to warrant some sort of publication. But what? Neither of us had any access to the "mainstream" media. Nor were we interested in seeking a book contract. We wanted to publish our findings in a form that would be cheap, accessible, and engaging for exactly the kind of women who had been our students at the College at Old Westbury, and this meant neither a book nor a magazine article. The decision we made, which now seems to us somewhat extraordinary, was to self-publish our results in booklet form. By self-publishing, we maintained control over the content, including the choice of illustrations and we had an inexpensive product that could easily be passed from hand to hand. We called our little vanity press Glass Mountain Pamphlets, referring to an obstacle—like sexism—that we might not yet be able to smash but could at least see through. Its headquarters was the house we shared with three other adults and Barbara's children.

The pamphlet was an instant success, at least as what the *Village Voice* called an "underground bestseller." Word of it spread through networks of women's groups as well as the through the countercultural underground newspapers of the time. Soon we found ourselves overwhelmed by the job of fulfilling orders—which we'd been shipping off in Pampers boxes generated by Barbara's infant son —and gratefully accepted the newly founded Feminist Press's offer to take over distribution. Eventually, *WMN* was translated into French, Spanish, German, Hebrew, Japanese, and Danish, and distributed in the UK. In 1993, one of us was invited to give a lecture tour in India, in part on the basis of the booklet's popularity there. We felt vindicated in our decision to self-publish as a booklet, which, according to the accounts of readers, was indeed being passed among hospital nurses and was to be found in the many women's bookstores and women's health clinics that sprang up in those times. In 1973, the Feminist Press also published a ninety-six page companion booklet, *Complaints and Disorders: The Sexual Politics of Sickness*, which describes the effects of solely male-defined medical expertise on nineteenth- and twentieth-century women.

Sometimes, when we consider the vast amounts of relevant scholarly research that has become available since the 1970s, we wish we could be starting this project all over again (although that would be impossible, since some of that new research was inspired in part by *WMN*!) There is now a wealth of information about women as lay healers, midwives, and "doctresses" in early America and their subsequent exclusion from formal medical education in the nineteenth and twentieth centuries. If anything, even more information has become available about women as lay healers in early modern Europe, and their fates in the witch persecutions of the time—enough to tempt us into what could be many rewarding years of study. Much of this work bolsters and fleshes out our assertions in *WMN*, but some of it requires that we update and correct the original text.

First, on the matter of the number of women killed as witches, we used the estimates available to us at the time—scholars accepted figures of one million or even much higher. Although the body count will never be exact, historian John Demos writes that recent studies yield estimates that "fall in a range of "50,000 to 100,000." Demos adds that, "These, in turn, were just a fraction of a much larger number of suspects. . . ."[1]

Second, we should clarify the role of the European medical profession relative to church and state. Witch trials represented extraordinary cooperation (and sometimes conflict) among all the dominant institutions, including both the legal and medical professions, which were heavily dependent on approval from the highest authorities. It was the medical profession that provided the courts with expert testimony: for example, Paulus Zacchias, the personal physician to two seventeenth-century Popes, authored a seven-volume treatise called *Medico-Legal Questions* to demonstrate "where medical knowledge could inform Canon Law on such issues as . . . the causes of foetal death, types of madness, poisoning, impotence, malingering, torture, [and] witchcraft . . ."[2]

Physicians benefited from the suppression of their competition: in the European cities where they congregated, they practiced in a market filled with lay healers and empirics. In London, in 1600, there were fifty physicians affiliated with the College of Physicians (a stronghold of Galenic medicine), outnumbered by some 250 mainly unlicensed practitioners (not including surgeons, apothecaries, midwives, and nurses) who a made a living.[3] In 1581, the College of Physicians, which claimed the right to regulate medical practice in London, attempted to prevent a lay healer named Margaret Kennix from practicing—but Queen Elizabeth had intervened, decreeing that "the poore woman should be permitted by you quietly to practice and mynister to the curing of diseases and woundes, by the means of certain Simples [herbal remedies] in the applying wherof it seemth God hath given her an especial knowledge, to the benefit of the poorer sort. . . ."[4] Such protection for her favored few was not to last after Elizabeth's death in 1602.

We stand by our assertion that male physicians were both more dangerous and less effective than female lay healers. Francis Bacon (1561–1626) himself a scientific originator, thought that "empirics and old women" were "more happy many times in their cures than learned physicians." The conservative philosopher Thomas Hobbes (1588–1679) concluded that he would "rather have the advice or take physic from an experienced old woman that had been at many sick people's bedsides, than from the learnedst but unexperienced physician."[5]

Third, we made the assumption that witches may have met in "covens" or other organized groups, and we referred to Margaret Murray when we said that "some writers speculate that these may have been occasions for pagan religious worship." Murray's research has since been discredited, and today most scholars seem to agree that the beliefs of women who were executed as witches cannot be differentiated from those of the rest of the population, and most were avowedly Christian. Some pagan religions or remnants did survive in places but the connection between this and women accused of witchcraft remains unclear.

Another point worth revisiting concerns the religious wars in the background of the witch hunts. We wrote: ". . . witch-healer's methods were as great a threat (to the Catholic Church, if not the Protestant) as her results, for the witch was an empiricist . . ." We can no more do justice here to the conflicts of the Reformation and Counter-Reformation than we could in a short booklet. But it should be noted that while Protestants fought the Roman Catholic Church, they tortured and executed witches too.

But if we do stand corrected on these points, a few scholars, it seems to us, have gone too far in the other direction, sometimes with a view to discrediting *WMN*. For example, in 1990, our work was described as "trail-blazing" by an Oxford-based scholar, David Harley—but not in a good way.[6] While agreeing that witches were often folk healers, he criticized us, based on a survey of convictions in England, Scotland, and New England, (data which was not available when we wrote) for exaggerating the proportion of *midwives* among convicted witches, saying we had maligned midwives and created "a multitude of imaginary martyrs for the modern women's health movement." Others, like art historian Jane Davidson of the University of Nevada, seemed to echo him without adding any new data to the argument and began to refer, even less plausibly, to "the myth of the persecuted witch-healer."[7]

It is true that the only primary source available to us at the time was the fifteenth-century witch-hunters' guidebook, *The Malleus Malificarum*, which proclaimed that "No one does more harm to the Catholic Church than midwives."[8] Even now, with all the archival data that has become available, it's impossible for scholars to offer statistically firm generalizations about the occupations of women accused of witchcraft: usually, the convicted person's occupation was not recorded.

Yet the association that witch hunters made between witches and midwives in Europe is inescapable. Based on archival research in Germany, Lyndal Roper documents several examples, finding for instance, in 1590, in the town of Nördlingin, that one midwife, Barbara Lierheimer, had angrily let it be known that the executioner "had ruined her livelihood by putting it about that she was a witch." Soon she was arrested, and after many contradictory denials and confessions, finally tortured to death. In Würtzburg in 1627, Roper tells us that a "crafty midwife" was listed among those condemned, and the scribe has added in the margin the comment, "The whole business comes from her." Much later in the seventeenth century, in Augsberg,

Roper found the pastor at Holy Cross Church had "no compunctions about saying the local midwife was a witch, and he flatly refused to baptize any children she brought to the altar."[9]

Whatever the number of convicted midwives, few historians would dispute the prevalence of lay healers among those accused of witchcraft. According to historian Brian P. Levack, "studies of witchcraft depositions in Switzerland, Austria, Schleswig-Holstein, England, Scotland, and New England reveal that many of those who were prosecuted for witchcraft were in fact wise-women."He writes that it was their prominence as "cooks, healers and midwives" that made women in general "vulnerable to the charge that they practiced harmful magic."[10]

But "harmful magic" was not the only kind of accusation: as we pointed out in the pamphlet, the practice of healing or "white witchcraft" was itself a sign of being a follower of Satan. William Perkins (1558–1602), an English Protestant minister and theologian, was one of the clergymen who introduced continental ideas of witchcraft into England and New England. He preached that in addition to "bad witches," there were "good witches" who only cured the "hurts" that had been inflicted by "bad witches," explaining: ". . . of the two the more horrible and detestable monster is the good witch . . . which are better known than the bad, being commonly called wisemen or wisewomen. This will appear by experience in most places in this country."[11]

In colonial New England, which we did not attempt to cover in *WMN*, recent scholarship has revealed much more about the relationship between healers and witch persecutions. According to David D. Hall, healers in seventeenth century New England seem to have been "especially vulnerable" to charges of witchcraft. Healing was considered suspicious because it "did not rely on confession of sin" to clergy, and disease was still thought to be caused by either God or the Devil.[12] In *The Enemy Within*, John Demos describes the profile of the typical woman tried for witchcraft in New England, writing that perhaps a quarter to a third of the suspect group was known for "making and administering special 'remedies,' providing expert forms of nursing, or serving in some regular way as midwives. A few were specifically described as 'doctor women.' . . . .The underlying linkage here is obvious enough; the ability to heal and the ability to harm seemed intimately related." Demos speculates about the general effect of the persecutions: "Clearly, the wisest course in early modern community life—especially for a woman—was to blend in and *not* to seem too openly self-assertive. To be, or to behave, otherwise was to open oneself to suspicion of witchcraft."[13]

Looking back after all these years, what strikes us about the witch hunts are not only the bizarre beliefs that inspired them and the personal tragedies that ensued, but the sheer waste of talent and knowledge that they represented. The victims, besides the individual women who were tortured and executed, were also all the people who were consequently deprived of their healing or midwifery skills. At a time we now associate with the Renaissance in Europe and the first signs of the scientific revolution, the witch hunts were a step back toward ignorance and helplessness—and not only for the largely lower-class people who lost so many of their traditional healers.

Instead, what could have been a proud occupation for women and a field for lively intellectual inquiry was discredited when not actually obliterated, so that later, when members of the educated elite sought to recapture some of the lost knowledge of the natural world, they had to turn to fairly marginal remnants of the old healing tradition. As Richard Holmes writes of the great English botanist Joseph Banks in the mid-eighteenth century, his interest in botany: ". . . brought him into contact with a race of people who would normally have been quite invisible to a privileged Eton schoolboy such as he. These were the wise women of the country lanes and hedgerows, the gypsy herbalists who collected "simples" or medicinal plants . . . They were a strange but knowledgeable tribe, whom he soon learned to treat with respect."[14]

The suppression of the "witches" and the later, less violent elimination of midwives and aspiring female doctors in the United States are hardly the only instances in history of willfully squandered talent, education, and experience. Human intellectual progress proceeds, to the extent that it does at all, only haltingly, with ghastly interruptions for the slaughter of suspicious individuals or groups, colonial extirpations of indigenous cultures, and backslidings into religiously imposed ignorance. Sometimes an important task for progressives is the "conservative" one of recovering, or at least pointing out, what was lost.

We are immensely proud of the role this little booklet has played in women's reclamation of healing roles in the late twentieth century—not all by itself of course, but along with the larger women's movement and women's health movement that it grew out of. It helped inspire young women to go to medical school, to recreate the profession of midwifery in America, and to advance the status of the nursing profession. We would underscore for new readers, however, that our concern was for class and racial equity as well as for women as a group. Compared to what we confronted in the 1970s, today's American health care system features far more women as practitioners and even decision makers, but it is also more single-mindedly driven by profit. We are hopeful that Obama's health reform will curb its murderous tendency to exclude those who most need care, but basic problems of access and affordability will remain. For all our gains, we clearly have our work cut out for us.

Barbara Ehrenreich
Deirdre English
March 2010

NOTES

1. John Demos, *The Enemy Within: 2000 Years of Witch-Hunting in the Western World* (New York: Viking, 2008), 38.

2. Andrew Wear, Lawrence I. Conrad, et al, *The Western Medical Tradition 800 bc–1800*, The Wellcome Institute for the History of Medicine (Cambridge: Cambridge University Press, 1995), 237.

3. *Ibid.*, 233.

4. *Ibid.*, 236.

5. Keith Thomas, *Religion and the Decline of Magic: Studies in Popular Beliefs in Sixteenth and Seventeenth Century England* (London: Weidenfeld and Nicolson, 1971), 14.

6. David Harley, *"Historians as Demonologists: The Myth of the Midwife-Witch," The Society for the Social History of Medicine* (1990): 1–26.

7. Jane P. Davidson, "The Myth of the Persecuted Female Healer," in *The Witchcraft Reader*, 2nd edition, ed. Darren Oldridge (New York: Routledge, 2008), 257.

8. Henricus Institoris, O.P. and Jacobus Sprenger, O.P., *The Malleus Maleficarum*, vol II, trans. and ed. Christopher S. MacKay (Cambridge: Cambridge University Press, 2006), 164.

9. Lyndal Roper, *Witch Craze* (New Haven and London: Yale University Press, 2004) 70, 33, 187.

10. Brian P. Levack, *The Witch-Hunt in Early Modern Europe, Third Edition* (Harlow, England: Pearson Longman, 1995), 146, 127.

11. William Perkins, "The Damned Art of Witchcraft," excerpted in *The Witchcraft Sourcebook* by Brian P. Levack (New York: Routledge, 2004), 94–6.

12. David D. Hall, *Witch Hunting in Seventeenth Century New England: A Documentary History 1638–1693* (Boston: Northeastern University Press, 1991), 5.

13. Demos, *The Enemy Within*, 119, 43.

14. Richard Holmes, *The Age of Wonder: How the Romantic Generation Discovered the Beauty and Terror of Science* (New York: Pantheon, 2008), 7.

Introduction to the First Edition

WOMEN HAVE ALWAYS BEEN HEALERS. THEY WERE THE unlicensed doctors and anatomists of Western history. They were abortionists, nurses, and counselors. They were pharmacists, cultivating healing herbs and exchanging secrets of their uses. They were midwives, travelling from home to home and village to village. For centuries women were doctors without degrees, barred from books and lectures, learning from each other, and passing on experience from neighbor to neighbor and mother to daughter. They were called "wise women" by the people, witches or charlatans by the authorities. Medicine is part of our heritage as women, our history, our birthright.

Today, however, health care is the property of male professionals. Ninety-three percent of the doctors in the US are men, as are almost all the top directors and administrators of health institutions. Women are still in the overall majority—70 percent of health workers are women—but we have been incorporated as *workers* into an industry where the bosses are men. We are no longer independent practitioners, known by our own names, for our own work. We are, for the most part, institutional fixtures filling faceless job slots: clerk, dietary aide, technician, maid.

When we are allowed to participate in the healing process, we can do so only as nurses. And nurses of every rank from aide up are just "ancillary workers" in relation to the doctors (from the Latin *ancilla*, maid servant). From the nurses' aide, whose menial tasks are spelled out with industrial precision, to the "professional" nurse, who translates the doctors' orders into the aide's tasks, nurses share the status of a uniformed maid service to the dominant male professionals.

Our subservience is reinforced by our ignorance, and our ignorance is *enforced.* Nurses are taught not to question, not to challenge. "The doctor knows best." He is the shaman, in touch with the forbidden, mystically complex world of Science which we have been taught is beyond our grasp. Women health workers are alienated from the scientific substance of their work, restricted to the "womanly" business of nurturing and housekeeping—a passive, silent majority.

We are told that our subservience is biologically ordained: women are inherently nurse-like and not doctor-like. Sometimes we even try to console ourselves with the theory that we *were* defeated by anatomy before we were defeated by men, that women have been so trapped by the cycles of menstruation and reproduction that they have never been free and creative agents outside their homes. Another myth, fostered by conventional medical histories, is that male professionals won out on the strength of their superior technology. According to these accounts, (male) science more or less automatically replaced (female) superstition—which from then on was called "old wives' tales."

But history belies these theories. Women have been autonomous healers, often the only healers for women and the poor. And we found, in the periods we have studied, that, if anything, it was the male professionals who clung to untested doctrines and ritualistic practices—and it was the women healers who represented a more human, empirical approach to healing.

Our position in the health system today is not "natural." It is a condition which has to be explained. In this pamphlet we have asked: How did we arrive at our present position of subservience from our former position of leadership?

We learned this much: the suppression of women health workers and the rise to dominance of male professionals was not a "natural" process, resulting automatically from changes in medical science, nor was it the result of women's failure to take on healing work. It was an active *takeover* by male professionals. And it was not science that enabled men to win out: the critical battles took place long before the development of modern scientific technology.

The stakes of the struggle were high: political and economic monopolization of medicine meant control over its institutional organizations, its theory and practice, its profits and prestige. And the stakes are even higher today, when total control of medicine means potential power to determine who will live and who will die, who is fertile and who is sterile, who is "mad" and who is sane.

The suppression of female healers by the medical establishment was a political struggle, first, in that it is part of the history of sex struggle in general. The status of women healers has risen and fallen with the status of women. When women healers were attacked, they were attacked as *women*; when they fought back, they fought back in solidarity with all women.

It was a political struggle, second, in that it was part of a *class* struggle. Women healers were people's doctors, and their medicine was part of a people's subculture. To this very day women's medical practices have thrived in the midst of rebellious lower-class movements which have struggled to be free from the established authorities. Male professionals, on the other hand, served the ruling class—both medically and politically. Their interests have been advanced by the universities, the philanthropic foundations, and the law. They owe their victory—not so much to their own efforts—but to the intervention of the ruling class they served.

This pamphlet represents a beginning of the research which will have to be done to recapture our history as health workers. It is a fragmentary account, assembled from sources that were usually sketchy and often biased, by women who are in no sense "professional" historians. We confined ourselves to Western history, since the institutions we confront today are the products of Western civilization. We are far from being able to present a complete chronological history. Instead, we looked at two separate, important phases in the male takeover of health care: the suppression of witches in medieval Europe, and the rise of the male medical profession in nineteenth century America.

To know our history is to begin to see how to take up the struggle again.

Witchcraft and Medicine in the Middle Ages

WITCHES LIVED AND WERE BURNED LONG BEFORE
the development of modern medical technology. The
great majority of them were lay healers serving the
peasant population, and their suppression marks one
of the opening struggles in the history of man's suppression of women as healers.

The other side of the suppression of witches as
healers was the creation of a new male medical profession, under the protection and patronage of the ruling
classes. This new European medical profession played
an important role in the witch hunts, supporting the
witches' persecutors with "medical" reasoning:

> . . . Because the Medieval Church, with the sup-
> port of kings, princes and secular authorities,

controlled medical education and practice, the Inquisition [witch hunts] constitutes, among other things, an early instance of the "professional" repudiating the skills and interfering with the rights of the "nonprofessional" to minister to the poor. (Thomas Szasz, *The Manufacture of Madness*)

The witch hunts left a lasting effect: an aspect of the female has ever since been associated with the witch, and an aura of contamination has remained—

Witch healing peasants (Breughel)

especially around the midwife and other women healers. This early and devastating exclusion of women
from independent healing roles was a violent prece-
dent and a warning: it was to become a theme of our
history. The women's health movement of today has
ancient roots in the medieval covens, and its opponents
have as their ancestors those who ruthlessly forced the
elimination of witches.

THE WITCH CRAZE

The age of witch hunting spanned more than four
centuries (from the fourteenth to the seventeenth century) in its sweep from Germany to England. It was
born in feudalism and lasted—gaining in virulence—
well into the "age of reason." The witch craze took different forms at different times and place, but never lost
its essential character: that of a ruling class campaign
of terror directed against the female peasant population. Witches represented a political, religious, and
sexual threat to the Protestant and Catholic churches
alike, as well as to the State.

The extent of the witch craze is startling: In the
late fifteenth and early sixteenth centuries there were
thousands upon thousands of executions—usually live
burnings at the stake—in Germany, Italy, and other

countries. In the mid-sixteenth century the terror spread to France, and finally to England. One writer has estimated the number of executions on an average of 600 a year for certain German cities—or two a day, "leaving out Sundays." Nine hundred witches were destroyed in a single year in the Wertzberg area, and 1000 in and around Como. At Toulouse, four hundred were put to death in a day. In the Bishopric of Trier, in 1585, two villages were left with only one female inhabitant each. Many writers have estimated the total number killed to have been in the millions.

Women made up some 85 percent of those executed—old women, young women, and children.*

Their scope alone suggests that the witch hunts represent a deep-seated social phenomenon which goes far beyond the history of medicine. In locale and timing, the most virulent witch hunts were associated with periods of great social upheaval shaking feudalism at its roots—mass peasant uprisings and conspiracies, the beginnings of capitalism, and the rise of Protestantism. There is fragmentary evidence—which feminists ought to follow up suggesting that in some areas witchcraft represented a female-led peasant rebellion. Here we can't attempt to explore the historical context of the witch hunts in any depth. But we do have to get beyond some common myths about the witch craze—myths that rob the "witch" of any dignity and put the blame on her and the peasants she served.

Unfortunately, the witch herself—poor and illiterate—did not leave us her story. It was recorded, like all history, by the educated elite, so that today we know the witch only through the eyes of her persecutors.

Two of the most common theories of the witch

*We are omitting from this discussion any mention of the New England witch trials in the 1600s. These trials occurred on a relatively small scale, very late in the history of witch hunts, and in an entirely different social context than the earlier European witch craze.

hunts are basically *medical* interpretations, attributing the witch craze to unexplainable outbreaks of mass hysteria. One version has it that the peasantry went mad. According to this, the witch craze was an epidemic of mass hatred and panic cast in images of a blood-lusty peasant mob bearing flaming torches. Another psychiatric interpretation holds that the witches themselves were insane. One authoritative psychiatric historian, Gregory Zilboorg, wrote that:

> . . . millions of witches, sorcerers, possessed and obsessed were an enormous mass of severe neurotics [and] psychotics . . . for many years the world looked like veritable insane asylum . . .

But, in fact, the witch craze was neither a lynching party nor a mass suicide by hysterical women. Rather, it followed well-ordered, legalistic procedures. The witch hunts were well-organized campaigns, initiated, financed, and executed by Church and State. To Catholic and Protestant witch hunters alike, the unquestioned authority on how to conduct a witch hunt was *The Malleus Maleficarum*, or *Hammer of Witches*, written in 1484 by the Reverends Kramer and Sprenger (the "beloved sons" of Pope Innocent VIII.) For three centuries this sadistic book lay on the bench of every

IOAN PRENTIS
& his Bid

JACKE
GILL

Three witches hanging, from the title page of a contemporary pamphlet on the third Chelmsford witch trial, 1589

judge, every witch hunter. In a long section on judicial proceedings, the instructions make it clear how the "hysteria" was set off: the job of initiating a witch trial was to be performed by either the Vicar (priest) or Judge of the County, who was to post a notice to

> direct, command, require and admonish that within the space of twelve days . . . that they should reveal it unto us if anyone know, see or have heard that any person is reported to be a heretic or a witch, or if any is suspected espe-

cially of such practices as cause injury to men, cattle, or the fruits of the earth, to the loss of the State.

Anyone failing to report a witch faced both excommunication and a long list of temporal punishments.

If this threatening notice exposed at least one witch, her trial could be used to unearth several more. Kramer and Sprenger gave detailed instructions about the use of torture to force confessions and further accusations. Commonly, the accused was stripped naked and shaved of all her body hair, then subjected to thumbscrews and the rack, spikes and bone-crushing "boots," starvation and beatings. The point is obvious: the witch craze did not arise spontaneously in the peasantry. It was a calculated ruling class campaign of terrorization.

THE CRIMES OF WITCHES

Who were the witches, then, and what were their "crimes" that could arouse such vicious upper-class suppression? Undoubtedly, over the centuries of witch hunting, the charge of "witchcraft" came to cover a multitude of sins ranging from political subversion and religious heresy to lewdness and blasphemy. But three central accusations emerge repeatedly in the history of witchcraft throughout northern Europe: First, witches are accused of every conceivable sexual crime against men. Quite simply, they are "accused" of female sexuality. Second, they are accused of being organized. Third, they are accused of having magical powers effecting health—of harming, but also of healing. They were often charged specifically with possessing medical and obstetrical skills.

First, consider the charge of sexual crimes. The

Devil seducing a witch

medieval Catholic Church elevated sexism to a point of principle: *The Malleus* declares, "When a woman thinks alone, she thinks evil." The misogyny of the Church, if not proved by the witch craze itself, is demonstrated by its teaching that in intercourse the male deposits in the female a homunculus, or "little person," complete with soul, which is simply housed in the womb for nine months, without acquiring any attributes of the mother. The homunculus is not really safe, however, until it reaches male hands again, when a priest baptises it, ensuring the salvation of its immortal soul. Another depressing fantasy of some medieval religious thinkers was that upon resurrection all human beings would be reborn as men!

The Church associated women with sex, and all

pleasure in sex was condemned, because it could only come from the devil. Witches were supposed to have gotten pleasure from copulation with the devil (despite the icy-cold organ he was reputed to possess) and they in turn infected men. Lust in either man or wife, then, was blamed on the female. On the other hand, witches were accused of making men impotent and of causing their penises to disappear. As for female sexuality, witches were accused, in effect, of giving contraceptive aid and of performing abortions:

> Now there are, as it is said in the Papal Bull, seven methods by which they infect with witch-craft the venereal act and the conception of the womb: First, by including the minds of men to inordinate passion; second, by obstructing their generative force; third, by removing the members accommodated to that act; fourth, by changing men into beasts by their magic act; fifth by destroying the generative force in women; sixth, by procuring abortion; seventh, by offering children to the devils, besides other animals and fruits of the earth with which they work much harm . . .
>
> (*The Malleus Maleficarum*)

In the eyes of the Church, all the witch's power was ultimately derived from her sexuality. Her career began with sexual intercourse with the devil. Each witch was confirmed at a general meeting (the witches' Sabbath) at which the devil presided, often in the form of a goat, and had intercourse with the neophytes. In return for her powers, the witch promised to serve him faithfully. (In the imagination of the Church even evil could only be thought of as ultimately male-directed!) As *The Malleus* makes clear, the devil almost always acts through the female, just as he did in Eden:

> All witchcraft comes from carnal lust, which in women is insatiable . . . Wherefore for the sake of fulfilling their lusts they consort with devils . . . it is sufficiently clear that it is no matter for wonder that there are more women than men found infected with the heresy of witchcraft . . . And blessed be the Highest Who has so far preserved the male sex from so great a crime . . .

Not only were the witches women—they were women who seemed to be organized into an enormous secret society. A witch who was proved member of the "Devil's party" was more dreadful than one who had acted alone, and the witch hunting literature is obsessed with the question of what went on at the witches' "Sabbaths." (Eating of unbaptised babies? Bestialism and mass orgies? So went their lurid speculations . . .)

In fact, there is evidence that women accused of being witches did meet locally in small groups and that these groups came together in crowds of hundreds or thousands on festival days. Some writers speculate that the meetings were occasions for pagan religious worship. Undoubtedly the meetings were also occasions for trading herbal lore and passing on the news.

Witches and demons dancing in a ring

We have little evidence about the political significance of the witches' organizations, but it's hard to imagine that they weren't connected to the peasant rebellions of the time. Any peasant organization, just by being an organization, would attract dissidents, increase communication between villages, and build a spirit of collectivity and autonomy among the peasants.

WITCHES AS HEALERS

We come now to the most fantastic accusation of all: the witch is accused not only of murdering and poisoning, sex crimes and conspiracy—but of *helping and healing*. As a leading English witch hunter put it:

> For this must always be remembered, as a conclusion, that by witches we understand not only those which kill and torment, but all Diviners, Charmers, Jugglers, all Wizards, commonly called wise men and wise women . . . and in the same number we reckon all good Witches, which do no hurt but good, which do not spoil and destroy, but save and deliver . . . It were a thousand times better for the land if all Witches, but especially the blessing Witch, might suffer death.

Witch-healers were often the only general medical practitioners for a people who had no doctors and no hospitals and who were bitterly afflicted with poverty and disease. In particular, the association of the witch and the midwife was strong: "No one does more harm to the Catholic Church than midwives," wrote witch hunters Kramer and Sprenger.

The Church itself had little to offer the suffering peasantry:

> On Sundays, after Mass, the sick came in scores, crying for help, - and words were all they got: "You have sinned, and God is afflicting you. Thank him; you will suffer so much less torment in the life to come. Endure, suffer, die. Has not the Church its prayers for the dead?"
>
> (Jules Michelet, *Satanism and Witchcraft*)

When faced with the misery of the poor, the Church turned to the dogma that experience in this world is fleeting and unimportant. But there was a double standard at work, for the Church was not against medical care for the upper class. Kings and nobles had their court physicians who were men, sometimes even priests. The real issue was control: male upper-class

Witch preparing a potion

healing under the auspices of the Church was acceptable, female healing as part of a peasant subculture was not.

The Church saw its attack on peasant healers as an attack on *magic*, not medicine. The devil was believed to have real power on earth, and the use of that power by peasant women—whether for good or evil—was frightening to the Church and State. The greater their satanic powers to help themselves, the less they were dependent on God and the Church, and the more they were potentially able to use their powers against God's order. Magic charms were thought to be at least as effective as prayer in healing the sick, but prayer was Church-sanctioned and controlled while incantations and charms were not. Thus magic cures, even when successful, were an accursed interference with the will of God, achieved with the help of the devil, and the cure itself was evil. There was no problem in distinguishing God's cures from the devil's, for obviously the Lord would work through priests and doctors rather than through peasant women.

The wise woman, or witch, had a host of remedies which had been tested in years of use. Many of the herbal remedies developed by witches still have their place in modern pharmacology. They had pain-killers, digestive aids, and anti-inflammatory agents. They used ergot for the pain of labor at a time when the Church held that pain in labor was the Lord's just punishments for Eve's original sin. Ergot derivatives are the principal drugs used today to hasten labor and aid in the recovery from childbirth. Belladonna—still used today as an anti-spasmodic—was used by the witch-healers to inhibit uterine contractions when miscarriage threatened. Digitalis, still an important drug in treating heart ailments, is said to have been discovered by an English witch. Undoubtedly many of the witches' other remedies were purely magical, and owed their effectiveness—if they had any—to their reputation.

The witch-healer's methods were as great a threat (to the Catholic Church, if not the Protestant) as her results, for the witch was an empiricist: she relied on her senses rather than on faith or doctrine, she believed in trial and error, cause and effect. Her attitude was not religiously passive, but actively inquiring. She trusted her ability to find ways to deal with disease, pregnancy, and childbirth—whether through medications or charms. In short, her magic was the science of her time.

The Church, by contrast, was deeply anti-empirical. It discredited the value of the material world, and had a profound distrust of the senses. There was no point in looking for natural laws that govern physical phenomena, for the world is created anew by God in every instant. Kramer and Sprenger, in *The Malleus*, quote St. Augustine on the deceptiveness of the senses:

> ... Now the motive of the will is something perceived through the senses or the intellect, both of which are subject to the power of the devil.

> For St. Augustine says in Book 83: This evil, which is of the devil, creeps in by all the sensual approaches; he places himself in figures, he adapts himself to colors, he attaches himself to sounds, he lurks in angry and wrongful conversation, he abides in smells, he impregnates with flavours and fills with certain exhalations all the channels of the understanding.

The senses are the devil's playground, the arena into which he will try to lure men away from Faith and into the conceits of the intellect or the delusions of carnality.

In the persecution of the witch, the anti-empiricist and the misogynist, anti-sexual obsessions of the Church coincide: empiricism and sexuality both represent a surrender to the senses, a betrayal of faith. The witch was a triple threat to the Church: She was a woman, and not ashamed of it. She appeared to be part of an organized underground of peasant women. She was a healer whose practice was based in empirical study. In the face of the repressive fatalism of Christianity, she held out the hope of change in this world.

THE RISE OF THE EUROPEAN
MEDICAL PROFESSION

While witches practiced among the people, the ruling classes were cultivating their own breed of secular healers: the university-trained physicians. In the
century that preceded the beginning of the "witch
craze"—the thirteenth century—European medicine
became firmly established as a secular science and a
profession. The medical profession was actively engaged
in the elimination of female healers—their exclusion
from the universities, for example—long before the
witch hunts began.

For eight long centuries, from the fifth to the
thirteenth, the otherworldly, anti-medical stance of
the Church has stood in the way of the development
of medicine as a respectable profession. Then, in the
thirteenth century, there was a revival of learning,
touched off by contact with the Arab world. Medical schools appeared in the universities, and more and
more young men of means sought medical training.
The church imposed strict controls on the new profession, and allowed it to develop only within the terms
set by Catholic doctrine. University-trained physicians were not permitted to practice without calling
in a priest to aid and advise them, or to treat a patient

who refused confession. By the fourteenth century their practice was in demand among the wealthy, as long as they continued to take pains to show that their attention to the body did not jeopardize the soul. In fact, accounts of their medical training make it seem more likely that they jeopardized the *body*.

There was nothing in late medieval medical training that conflicted with church doctrine, and little that we would recognize as "science." Medical students, like other scholarly young gentlemen, spent years studying Plato, Aristotle, and Christian theology. Their medical theory was largely restricted to the works of Galen, the ancient Roman physician who stressed the theory of "complexions" or "temperaments" of men, "wherefore the choleric are wrathful, the sanguine are kindly, the melancholy are envious," and so on. While a

The humors: sanguine, melancholy, hot-tempered, sluggish

student, a doctor rarely saw any patients at all, and no experimentation of any kind was taught. Medicine was sharply differentiated from surgery, which was almost everywhere considered a degrading, menial craft, and the dissection of bodies was almost unheard of.

Confronted with a sick person, the university-trained physician had little to go on but superstition. Bleeding was a common practice, especially in the case of wounds. Leeches were applied according to the time, the hour, the air, and other similar considerations. Medical theories were often grounded more in "logic" than in observation: "Some food brought on good humors, and others, evil humours. For example, nasturtium, mustard, and garlic produced reddish bile; lentils, cabbage and the meat of old goats and beeves begot black bile." Incantations, and quasi-religious rituals were thought to be effective: the physician to Edward II, who held a bachelor's degree in theology and a doctorate in medicine from Oxford, prescribed for toothache writing on the jaws of a patient, "In the name of the Father, the Son, and the Holy Ghost, Amen," or touching a needle to a caterpillar and then to the tooth. A frequent treatment for leprosy was a broth made of the flesh of a black snake caught in a dry land among stones.

Such was the state of medical "science" at the time

The benefits of bleeding

when witch-healers were persecuted for being practitioners of "magic." It was witches who developed an extensive understanding of bones and muscles, herbs and drugs, while physicians were still deriving their prognoses from astrology and alchemists were trying to turn lead into gold. So great was the witches' knowledge that in 1527, Paracelsus, considered the "father of modern medicine," burned his text on pharmaceuticals, confessing that he "had learned from the Sorceress all he knew."

THE SUPPRESSION OF WOMEN HEALERS

The establishment of medicine as a profession, requiring university training, made it easy to bar women legally from practice. With few exceptions, the universities were closed to women (even to upper-class women who could afford them), and licensing laws were established to prohibit all but university-trained doctors from practice. It was impossible to enforce the licensing laws consistently since there were only a handful of university-trained doctors compared to the great mass of lay healers. But the laws *could* be used selectively. Their first target was not the peasant healer, but the better off, literate woman healer who competed for the same urban clientele as that of the university-trained doctors.

Take, for example, the case of Jacoba Felicie, brought to trial in 1322 by the Faculty of Medicine at the University of Paris, on charges of illegal practice. Jacoba was literate and had received some unspecified "special training" in medicine. That her patients were well off is evident from the fact that (as they testified in court) they had consulted well-known university-trained physicians before turning to her. The primary accusations brought against her were that

> . . . she would cure her patient of internal illness and wounds or of external abscesses. She would visit the sick assiduously and continue to examine the urine in the manner of physicians, feel the pulse, and touch the body and limbs.

Six witnesses affirmed that Jacoba had cured them, even after numerous doctors had given up, and one patient declared that she was wiser in the art of surgery and medicine than any master physician or surgeon in Paris. But these testimonials were used against her, for the charge was not that she was incompetent, but that—as a woman—she dared to cure at all.

Along the same lines, English physicians sent a petition to Parliament bewailing the "worthless and presumptuous women who usurped the profession" and asking the imposition of fines and "long imprisonment" on any woman who attempted to "use the practyse of Fisyk." By the fourteenth century, the medical profession's campaign against urban, educated women

Woman treating dislocated jaw

healers was virtually complete throughout Europe. Male doctors had won a clear monopoly over the practice of medicine among the upper classes (except for obstetrics, which remained the province of female midwives even among the upper classes for another three centuries). They were ready to take on a key role in the elimination of the great mass of female healers—the "witches."

The partnership between Church, State, and medical profession reached full bloom in the witch trials. The doctor was held up as the medical "expert," giving an aura of science to the whole proceeding. He was asked to make judgments about whether certain women were witches and whether certain afflictions had been caused by witchcraft. *The Malleus* says: "And if it is asked how it is possible to distinguish whether an illness is caused by witchcraft or by some natural physical defect, we answer that the first [way] is by means of the *judgment of doctors . . .* " [Emphasis added]. In the witch hunts, the Church explicitly legitimized the doctors' professionalism, denouncing non-professional healing as equivalent to heresy: "If a woman dare to cure *without having studied* she is a witch and must die." (Of course, there wasn't any way for a woman to study.) Finally, the witch craze provided a handy excuse for the doctor's failings in every-day practice: Anything he couldn't cure was obviously the result of sorcery.

The distinction between "female" superstition and "male" medicine was made final by the very roles of the doctor and the witch at the trial. The trial in one stroke established the male physician on a moral and intellectual plane vastly above the female healer he was called to judge. It placed him on the side of God and Law, a professional on par with lawyers and theologians, while it placed her on the side of darkness, evil, and magic. He owed his new status not to medical or scientific achievements of his own, but to the Church and State he served so well.

THE AFTERMATH

Witch hunts did not eliminate the lower-class woman healer, but they branded her forever as superstitious and possibly malevolent. So thoroughly was she discredited among the emerging middle classes that in the seventeenth and eighteenth centuries it was possible for male practitioners to make serious inroads into that last preserve of female healing—midwifery. Non-professional male practitioners—"barber-surgeons"—

The lady as physician

led the assault in England, claiming technical superiority on the basis of their use of the obstetrical forceps. (The forceps were legally classified as a surgical instrument, and women were legally barred from surgical practice.) In the hands of the barber-surgeons, obstetrical practice among the middle class was quickly transformed from a neighborly service into a lucrative business, which real physicians entered in force in the eighteenth century. Female midwives in England organized and charged the male intruders with commercialism and dangerous misuse of the forceps. But it was too late—the women were easily put down as ignorant "old wives" clinging to the superstitions of the past.

Doctor delivering under a sheet, for modesty's sake

Women and the Rise of the American Medical Profession

IN THE US THE MALE TAKEOVER OF HEALING ROLES started later than in England or France, but ultimately went much further. There is probably no industrialized country with a lower percentage of women doctors than the US today: England has 24 percent; Russia has 75 percent; the US has only 7 percent. And while midwifery—*female* midwifery—is still a thriving occupation in Scandinavia, the United Kingdom, the Netherlands, etc., it has been virtually outlawed here since the early twentieth century. By the turn of the century, medicine here was closed to all but a tiny minority of necessarily tough and well-heeled women. What was left was nursing, and this was in no way a substitute for the autonomous roles women had enjoyed as midwives and general healers.

The question is not so much how women got "left out" of medicine and left with nursing, but how did these categories arise at all? To put it another way: How did one particular set of healers, who happened to be male, white, and middle class, manage to oust all the competing folk healers, midwives, and other practitioners who had dominated the American medical scene in the early 1800s?

The conventional answer given by medical historians is, of course, that there always was one *true* American medical profession—a small band of men whose scientific and moral authority flowed in an unbroken stream from Hippocrates, Galen, and the great European medical scholars. In frontier America these doctors had to combat, not only the routine problems of sickness and death, but the abuses of a host of lay practitioners—usually depicted as women, ex-slaves, Indians, and drunken patent medicine salesmen. Fortunately for the medical profession, in the late nineteenth century the American public suddenly developed a healthy respect for doctors' scientific knowledge, outgrew its earlier faith in quacks, and granted the true medical profession a lasting monopoly of the healing arts.

But the real answer is not in this made-up drama of science versus ignorance and superstition. It's part of the nineteenth century's long story of class and sex struggles for power in all areas of life. When women had a place in medicine, it was in a *people's* medicine. When that people's medicine was destroyed, there was no place for women—except in the subservient role of nurses. The set of healers who became *the* medical profession was distinguished not so much by its associations with modern science as by its associations with the emerging American business establishment. With all due respect to Pasteur, Koch, and the other great European medical researchers of the nineteenth century, it was the Carnegies and Rockefellers who intervened to secure the final victory of the American medical profession.

The US in 1800 could hardly have been a more unpromising environment for the development of a medical profession, or any profession, for that matter. Few formally trained physicians had emigrated here from Europe. There were very few schools of medicine in America and very few institutions of higher learning altogether. The general public, fresh from a war of national liberation, was hostile to professionalism and "foreign" elitisms of any type.

In Western Europe, university-trained physicians already had a centuries' old monopoly over the right to heal. But in America, medical practice was traditionally open to anyone who could demonstrate healing skills—regardless of formal training, race, or sex. Ann Hutchinson, the dissenting religious leader of the 1600s, was a practitioner of "general physik," as were many other ministers and their wives. The medical historian Joseph Kett reports that "one of the most respected medical men in late eighteenth century Windsor, Connecticut, for example, was a freed Negro called 'Dr. Primus.' In New Jersey, medical practice, except in extraordinary cases, was mainly in the hands of women as late as 1818 . . . "

"Regular" doctors try water treatment

Women frequently went into joint practices with their husbands: The husband handling the surgery, the wife the midwifery and gynecology, and everything else shared. Or a woman might go into practice after developing skills through caring for family members or through an apprenticeship with a relative or other established healer. For example, Harriet Hunt, one of America's first trained female doctors, became interested in medicine during her sister's illness, worked for a while with a husband-wife "doctor" team, then simply hung out her own shingle. (Only later did she undertake formal training.)

ENTER THE DOCTOR

In the early 1800s there was also a growing number of formally trained doctors who took great pains to distinguish themselves from the host of lay practitioners. The most important real distinction was that the formally trained, or "regular" doctors as they called themselves, were male, usually middle class, and almost always more expensive than the lay competition. The "regulars'" practices were largely confined to middle- and upper-class people who could afford the prestige of being treated by a "gentleman" of their own class. By 1800, fashion even dictated that upper- and middle-class women employ male "regular" doctors for obstetrical care—a custom which plainer people regarded as grossly indecent.

In terms of medical skills and theory, the so-called "regulars" had nothing to recommend them over the lay practitioners. Their "formal training" meant little even by European standards of the time: medical programs varied in length from a few months to two years; many medical schools had no clinical facilities; high school diplomas were not required for admission to medical schools. Not that serious academic training would have helped much anyway—there was no body of medical science to be trained in. Instead, the "regulars" were taught to treat most ills by "heroic" measures: massive bleeding, huge doses of laxatives, calomel (a laxative containing mercury) and, later, opium. (The European medical profession had little better to offer at this time either.) There is no doubt that their "cures" were often either fatal or more injurious than the original disease. In the judgment of Oliver Wendell Holmes, Sr., himself a distinguished physician, if all the medicines used by the "regular" doctors in the US were thrown into the ocean, it would be so much the better for mankind and so much the worse for the fishes.

Gynecological exam

The lay practitioners were undoubtedly safer and more effective than the "regulars." They preferred mild herbal medications, dietary changes, and hand-holding to heroic interventions. Maybe they didn't know any more than the "regulars," but at least they were less likely to do the patient harm. Left alone, they might well have displaced the "regular" doctors with even middle-class consumers in time. But they didn't know the right people. The "regulars," with their close ties to the upper class, had legislative clout. By 1830, thirteen states had passed medical licensing laws outlawing "irregular" practice and establishing the "regulars" as the only legal healers.

It was a premature move. There was no popular support for the idea of medical professionalism, much less for the particular set of healers who claimed it. And there was no way to enforce the new laws: The trusted healers of the common people could not be just legislated out of practice. Worse still—for the "regulars"—this early grab for medical monopoly inspired mass indignation in the form of a radical, popular health movement which came close to smashing medical elitism in America once and for all.

THE POPULAR HEALTH MOVEMENT

The Popular Health Movement of the 1830s and 40s is usually dismissed in conventional medical histories as the high-tide of quackery and medical cultism. In reality it was the medical front of a general social upheaval stirred up by feminist and working class movements. Women were the backbone of the Popular Health Movement. "Ladies Physiological Societies," the equivalent of our know-your-body courses, sprang up everywhere, bringing rapt audiences simple instruction in anatomy and personal hygiene. The emphasis was on preventive care, as opposed to the murderous "cures" practiced by the "regular" doctors. The Movement ran up the banner for frequent bathing (regarded as a vice by many "regular" doctors of the time), loose-fitting female clothing, whole grain cereals, temperance, and a host of other issues women could relate to. And, at about the time that Margaret Sanger's mother was a little girl, some elements of the Movement were already pushing birth control.

The Movement was a radical assault on medical elitism, and an affirmation of the traditional people's medicine. "Every man his own doctor," was the slogan of one wing of the Movement, and they made it very clear that they meant every woman too. The "regular," licensed doctors were attacked as members of the "parasitic, non-producing classes," who survived only because of the upper-class's "lurid taste" for calomel and bleeding. Universities (where the elite of the "regular" doctors were trained) were denounced as places where students "learn to look upon labor as servile and demeaning" and to identify with the upper class. Working-class radicals rallied to the cause, linking "King-craft, Priest-craft, Lawyer-craft and Doctor-craft" as the four great evils of the time. In New York State, the Movement was represented in the legislature by a member of the Workingman's Party, who took every opportunity to assail the "privileged doctors."

The "regular" doctors quickly found themselves outnumbered and cornered. From the left wing of the Popular Health Movement came a total rejection of "doctoring" as a paid occupation—much less an overpaid "profession." From the moderate wing came a host of new medical philosophies, or sects, to compete with the "regulars" on their own terms: eclecticism, Grahamism, homeopathy, plus many minor ones. The new sects set up their own medical schools, (emphasizing preventive care and mild herbal cures), and started graduating their own doctors. In this context of medical ferment, the old "regulars" began to look like just another sect, a sect whose particular philosophy happened to learn toward calomel, bleeding, and the other standbys of "heroic" medicine. It was impossible to tell who were the "real" doctors, and by the 1840s, medical licensing laws had been repealed in almost all of the states.

THE COMING RACE

Doctor Evangeline. 'BY THE BYE, MR SAWYER, ARE YOU ENGAGED TOMORROW AFTERNOON? I HAVE RATHER A TICKLISH OPERATION TO PERFORM—AN AMPUTATION, YOU KNOW.'

Mr Sawyer. 'I SHALL BE VERY HAPPY TO DO IT FOR YOU.'

Dr Evangeline. 'O, NO, NOT *THAT*! BUT WILL YOU KINDLY COME AND ADMINISTER THE CHLOROFORM FOR ME?'   *14.9.1872*

The peak of the Popular Health Movement coincided with the beginnings of an organized feminist movement, and the two were so closely linked that it's hard to tell where one began and the other left off. "This crusade for women's health [the Popular Health Movement] was related both in cause and effect to the demand for women's rights in general, and the health and feminist movements become indistinguishable at this point," according to Richard Shryock, the well-known medical historian. The Health Movement was concerned with women's rights in general, and the women's movement was particularly concerned with health and with women's access to medical training.

In fact, leaders of both groups used the prevailing sex stereotypes to argue that women were even better equipped to be doctors than men. "We cannot deny that women possess superior capacities for the science of medicine," wrote Samuel Thomson, a Health Movement leader, in 1834. (However, he felt surgery and the care of males should be reserved for male practitioners.) Feminists, like Sarah Hale, went further, claiming in 1852: "Talk about this [medicine] being the appropriate sphere for man and his alone! With tenfold more plausibility and reason we say it is the appropriate sphere for woman, and hers alone."

The new medical sects' schools did, in fact, open their doors to women at a time when "regular" medical training was all but closed to them. For example, Harriet Hunt was denied admission to Harvard Medical College, and instead went to a sectarian school for her formal training. (Actually, the Harvard faculty had voted to admit her—along with some black male students—but the students threatened to riot if they came.) The "regular" physicians could take the credit for training Elizabeth Blackwell, America's first female "regular," but her alma mater (a small school in upstate New York) quickly passed a resolution barring further female students. The first generally co-ed medical school was the "irregular" Eclectic Central Medical College of New York, in Syracuse. Finally, the first two all-female medical colleges, one in Boston and one in Philadelphia, were themselves "irregular."

Feminist researchers should really find out more about the Popular Health Movement. From the perspective of our movement today, it's probably more relevant than the women's suffrage struggle. To us, the most tantalizing aspects of the Movement are: (1) That it represented both class struggle and feminist struggle: Today, it's stylish in some quarters to write off purely feminist issues as middle-class concerns.

But in the Popular Health Movement we see a coming together of feminist and working-class energies. Is this because the Popular Health Movement naturally attracted dissidents of all kinds, or was there some deeper identity of purpose? (2) The Popular Health Movement was not just a movement for more and better medical care, but for a radically different kind of health care: it was a substantive challenge to the prevailing medical dogma, practice, and theory. Today we tend to confine our critiques to the organization of medical care, and assume that the scientific substratum of medicine is unassailable. We too should be developing the capability for the critical study of medical "science"—at least as it relates to women.

DOCTORS ON THE OFFENSIVE

At its height in the 1830s and 1840s, the Popular Health Movement had the "regular" doctors—the professional ancestors of today's physicians—running scared. Later in the nineteenth century, as the grassroots energy ebbed and the Movement degenerated into a set of competing sects, the "regulars" went back on the offensive. In 1848, they pulled together their first national organization, pretentiously named *the American* Medical Association (AMA). County and

32. Dr. Meilanion Jones, finding himself outstripped in the race for patients by the fair Doctoress Atalanta Robinson, gallantly throws her a wedding ring and wins the day.
Punch Almanack 1877

state medical societies, many of which had practically disbanded during the height of medical anarchy in the 30s and 40s, began to reform.

Throughout the latter part of the nineteenth century, the "regulars" relentlessly attacked lay practitioners, sectarian doctors, and women practitioners in general. The attacks were linked: women practitioners could be attacked because of their sectarian leanings; sects could be attacked because of their openness to women. The arguments against women doctors ranged from paternalistic (how could a respectable woman travel at night to a medical emergence?) to the hardcore sexist. In his presidential address to the AMA in 1871, Dr. Alfred Stille, said:

> Certain women seek to rival men in manly sports . . . and the strongminded ape them in all things, even in dress. In doing so they may command a sort of admiration such as all monstrous productions inspire, especially when they aim towards a higher type than their own.

The virulence of the American sexist opposition to women in medicine has no parallel in Europe. This is probably because: First, fewer European women were aspiring to medical careers at this time. Second, feminist movements were nowhere as strong as in the US, and here the male doctors rightly associated the entrance of women into medicine with organized feminism. And, third, the European medical profession was already more firmly established and hence less afraid of competition.

The rare woman who did make it into a "regular" medical school faced one sexist hurdle after another. There was the continuous harassment—often lewd—by the male students. There were professors who wouldn't discuss anatomy with a lady present. There were textbooks like a well-known 1848 obstetrical text which stated, "She [Woman] has a head almost too small for intellect but just big enough for love." There were respectable gynecological theories of the injurious effects of intellectual activity on the female reproductive organs.

Having completed her academic work, the would-be woman doctor usually found the next steps blocked. Hospitals were usually closed to women doctors, and even if they weren't, the internships were not open to women. If she did finally make it into practice, she found her brother "regulars" unwilling to refer patients to her and absolutely opposed to her membership in their medical societies.

And so it is all the stranger to us, and all the sadder, that what we might call the "women's health movement" began, in the late nineteenth century, to dissociate itself from its Popular Health Movement past and to strive for respectability. Members of irregular sects were purged from the faculties of the women's medical colleges. Female medical leaders such as Elizabeth Blackwell joined male "regulars" in demanding an end to lay midwifery and "a complete medical education" for all who practiced obstetrics. All this at a time when the "regulars" still had little or no "scientific" advantage over the sect doctors or lay healers.

The explanation, we suppose, was that the women who were likely to seek formal medical training at this

Medical diploma mill

time were middle class. They must have found it easier to identify with the middle-class "regular" doctors than with lower-class women healers or with the sectarian medical groups (which had earlier been identified with radical movements.) The shift in allegiance was probably made all the easier by the fact that, in the cities, female lay practitioners were increasingly likely to be immigrants. (At the same time, the possibilities for a cross-class women's movement on *any* issue were vanishing as working-class women went into the factories and middle-class women settled into Victorian ladyhood.) Whatever the exact explanation, the result was that middle-class women had given up the substantive attack on male medicine, and accepted the terms set by the emerging male medical profession.

PROFESSIONAL VICTORY

The "regulars" were still in no condition to make another bid for medical monopoly. For one thing, they still couldn't claim to have any uniquely effective methods or special body of knowledge. Besides, an occupational group doesn't gain a professional monopoly on the basis of technical superiority alone. A recognized profession is not just a group of self-proclaimed experts; it is a group which has authority *in the law* to select its own members and regulate their practice, i.e., to monopolize a certain field without outside interference. How does a particular group gain full professional status? In the words of sociologist Elliot Freidson:

> A profession attains and maintains its position by virtue of the protection and patronage of some elite segment of society which has been persuaded that there is some special value in its work.

In other words, professions are the creation of a ruling class. To become *the* medical profession, the "regular" doctors needed, above all, ruling class patronage.

By a lucky coincidence for the "regulars," both the science and the patronage became available around the same time, at the turn of the century. French and especially German scientists brought forth the germ theory of disease which provided, for the first time in human history, a rational basis for disease prevention and therapy. While the run-of-the-mill American doctor was still mumbling about "humors" and dosing people with calomel, a tiny medical elite was travelling to German universities to learn the new science. They returned to the US filled with reformist zeal. In 1893 German-trained doctors (funded by local philanthropists) set up the first American German-style medical school, Johns Hopkins.

As far as curriculum was concerned, the big innovation at Hopkins was integrating lab work in basic science with expanded clinical training. Other reforms included hiring full-time faculty, emphasizing research, and closely associating the medical school with a full university. Johns Hopkins also introduced the modern pattern of medical education—four years of medical school following four years of college—which of course barred most working class and poor people from the possibility of a medical education.

Meanwhile the US was emerging as the industrial leader of the world. Fortunes built on oil, coal, and the ruthless exploitation of American workers were maturing into financial empires. For the first time in American history, there were sufficient concentrations of corporate wealth to allow for massive, organized philanthropy, i.e., organized ruling-class intervention in the social, cultural, and political life of the nation. Foundations were created as the lasting instruments of this intervention—the Rockefeller and Carnegie foundations appeared in the first decade of the twentieth century. One of the earliest and highest items on their agenda was medical "reform," the creation of a respectable, scientific American medical profession.

The group of American medical practitioners that the foundations chose to put their money behind was, naturally enough, the scientific elite of the "regular" doctors. (Many of these men were themselves ruling class, and all were urbane, university-trained gentlemen.) Starting in 1903, foundation money began to pour into medical schools by the millions. The conditions were clear: conform to the Johns Hopkins model or close. To get the message across, the Carnegie Corporation sent a staff man, Abraham Flexner, out on a national tour of medical schools—from Harvard right down to the last third-rate commercial schools.

Flexner almost singlehandedly decided which schools would get the money—and hence survive. For the bigger and better schools (i.e, those which already had enough money to begin to institute the prescribed reforms), there was the promise of fat foundation grants. Harvard was one of the lucky winners, and its president could say smugly in 1907, "Gentlemen, the way to get endowments for medicine is to improve medical education." As for the smaller, poorer schools, which included most of the sectarian schools and special schools for blacks and women—Flexner did not consider them worth saving. Their options were to close, or to remain open and face public denunciation in the report Flexner was preparing.

The Flexner Report, published in 1910, was the foundations' ultimatum to American medicine. In its wake, medical schools closed by the score, including six of America's eight black medical schools and the majority of the "irregular" schools which had been a haven for female students. Medicine was established once and for all as a branch of "higher" learning, accessible only through lengthy and expensive university training. It's certainly true that as medical knowledge grew, lengthier training did become necessary. But Flexner and the foundation had no intention of making such training available to the great mass of lay healers and "irregular" doctors. Instead, doors were slammed shut to blacks, to the majority of women, and to poor, white men. (Flexner in his report bewailed the fact that any "crude boy or jaded clerk" had been able to seek medical training.) Medicine had become a white, male, middle-class occupation.

But it was more than an occupation. It had become, at last, a profession. To be more precise, one particular group of healers, the "regular" doctors, was now *the* medical profession. Their victory was not based on any skills of their own: The run-of-the-mill "regular" doctor did not suddenly acquire a knowledge of medical science with the publication of the Flexner Report. But he did acquire the *mystique* of science. So what if his own alma mater had been condemned in the Flexner Report; wasn't he a member of the AMA, and wasn't it in the forefront of scientific reform? The doctor had become—thanks to some foreign scientists and eastern foundations—the "man of science": beyond criticism, beyond regulation, very nearly beyond competition.

OUTLAWING THE MIDWIVES

In state after state, new, tough, licensing laws sealed the doctor's monopoly on medical practice. All that was left was to drive out the last holdouts of the old people's medicine—the midwives. In 1910, about 50 percent of all babies were delivered by midwives—most were blacks or working class immigrants. It was an intolerable situation to the newly emerging obstetrical specialty: For one thing, every poor woman who went to a midwife was one more case lost to academic teaching and research. America's vast lower class resources of obstetrical "teaching material" were being wasted on ignorant midwives. Besides which, poor women were spending an estimated five million dollars a year on midwives—five million dollars which could have been going to "professionals."

Publicly, however, the obstetricians launched their attacks on midwives in the name of science and reform. Midwives were ridiculed as "hopelessly dirty, ignorant, and incompetent." Specifically, they were held responsible for the prevalence of puerperal sepsis (uterine infections) and neonatal ophthalmia (blindness due to parental infection with gonorrhea). Both conditions were easily preventable by techniques well within the grasp of the least literate midwife (hand-washing for puerperal sepsis, and eye drops for the ophthalmia.) So the obvious solution for a truly public-spirited obstetrical profession would have been to make the appropriate preventive techniques known and available to the mass of midwives. This is in fact what happened in England, Germany, and most other European nations: Midwifery was upgraded through training to become an established, independent occupation.

But the American obstetricians had no real commitment to improved obstetrical care. In fact, a study by a Johns Hopkins professor in 1912 indicated that most American doctors were *less* competent than the midwives. Not only were the doctors themselves unreliable about preventing sepsis and ophthalmia but they also tended to be too ready to use surgical techniques which endangered mother or child. If anyone, then, deserved a legal monopoly on obstetrical care, it was the midwives, not the MD's. But the doctors had power, the midwives didn't. Under intense pressure from the medical profession, state after state passed laws outlawing midwifery and restricting the practice of obstetrics to doctors. For poor and working-class women, this actually meant worse—or no—obstetrical care. (For instance, a study of infant mortality rates in Washington showed an increase in infant mortality in the years immediately following the passage of the law forbidding midwifery.) For the new, male medical profession, the ban on midwives meant one less source of competition. Women had been routed from their last foothold as independent practitioners.

THE LADY WITH THE LAMP

The only remaining occupation for women in health was nursing. Nursing had not always existed as a paid occupation—it had to be invented. In the early nineteenth century, a "nurse" was simply a woman who happened to be nursing someone—a sick child or an

SHE BECOMES A TRAINED NURSE

aging relative. There were hospitals, and they did employ nurses. But the hospitals of the time served largely as refuges for the dying poor, with only token care provided. Hospital nurses, history has it, were a disreputable lot, prone to drunkenness, prostitution, and thievery. And conditions in the hospitals were often scandalous. In the late 1870s a committee investigating New York's Bellevue Hospital could not find a bar of soap on the premises.

If nursing was not exactly an attractive field to women workers, it was a wide open arena for women *reformers*. To reform hospital care, you had to reform nursing, and to make nursing acceptable to doctors and to women of "good character," it had to be given a completely new image. Florence Nightingale got her change in the battlefront hospitals of the Crimean War, where she replaced the old camp-follower "nurses" with a bevy of disciplined, sober, middle-aged ladies. Dorothea Dix, an American hospital reformer, introduced the new breed of nurses in the Union hospitals of the Civil War.

The new nurse—"the lady with the lamp," selflessly tending the wounded—caught the popular imagination. Real nursing school began to appear in England right after the Crimean War, and in the US right after the Civil War. At the same time, the number of hospitals began to increase to keep pace with the needs of medical education. Medical students needed hospitals to train in; good hospitals, as the doctors were learning, needed good nurses.

In fact, the first American nursing schools did their best to recruit actual upper-class women as students. Miss Euphemia Van Rensselear, of an old aristocratic New York family, graced Bellevue's first class. And at Johns Hopkins, where Isabel Hampton trained nurses at the University Hospital, a leading doctor could only complain that:

Miss Hampton has been most successful in getting probationers [students] of the upper class;

but unfortunately, she selects them altogether for their good looks and the House staff is by this time in a sad state.

Let us look a little more closely at the women who invented nursing, because, in a very real sense, nursing as we know it today is the product of their oppression as upper-class Victorian women. Dorothea Dix was an heiress of substantial means. Florence Nightingale and Louisa Schuyler (the moving force behind the creation of America's first Nightingale-style nursing school) were genuine aristocrats. They were refugees from the enforced leisure of Victorian ladyhood. Dix and Nightingale did not begin to carve out their reform careers until they were in their thirties, and faced with the prospect of a long, useless spinsterhood. They focused their energies on the care of the sick because this was a "natural" and acceptable interest for ladies of their class.

Nightingale and her immediate disciples left nursing with the indelible stamp of their own class biases. Training emphasized character, not skills. The finished product, the Nightingale nurse, was simply the ideal Lady, transplanted from home to the hospital, and absolved of reproductive responsibilities. To the doctor, she brought the wifely virtue of absolute obedience. To the patient, she brought the selfless devotion of a mother. To the lower level hospital employees, she brought the firm but kindly discipline of a household manager accustomed to dealing with servants.

But, despite the glamorous "lady with the lamp" image, most of nursing work was just low-paid, heavy-duty housework. Before long, most nursing schools were attracting only women from working-class and lower-middle-class homes, whose only other options were factory or clerical work. But the philosophy of nursing education did not change—after all, the educators were still middle and upper-class women. If anything, they toughened their insistence on lady-like character development, and the socialization of nurses became what it has been for most of the twentieth century: the imposition of upper-class cultural values on working-class women. (For example, until recently, most nursing students were taught such upper-class graces as tea pouring, art appreciation, etc. Practical nurses are still taught to wear girdles, use make-up, and in general mimic the behavior of a "better" class of women.)

But the Nightingale nurse was not just the projection of upper-class ladyhood onto the working world: She embodied the very spirit of femininity as defined by sexist Victorian society—she was Woman. The inventors of nursing saw it as a natural vocation for women, second only to motherhood. When a group of English nurses proposed that nursing model itself after the medical profession, with exams and licensing, Nightingale responded that " . . . nurses cannot be registered and examined *any more than mothers.*" [Emphasis added.] Or, as one historian of nursing put it, nearly a century later, "Woman is an instinctive nurse, taught by Mother Nature." (Victor Robinson, MD, *White Caps, The Story of Nursing*). If women were instinctive nurses, they were not, in the Nightingale view, instinctive doctors. She wrote of the few female physicians of her time: "They have only tried to be men, and they have succeeded only in being third-rate men." Indeed, as the number of nursing students rose in the late-nineteenth century, the number of female medical students began to decline. Woman had found her place in the health system.

Just as the feminist movement had not opposed the rise of medical professionalism, it did not challenge nursing as an oppressive female role. In fact, feminists of the late-nineteenth century were themselves beginning to celebrate the nurse/mother image of femininity. The American women's movement had given up the struggle for full sexual equality to focus exclusively on the vote, and to get it, they were ready to adopt the most sexist tenets of Victorian ideology: Women need the vote, they argued, not because they are human, but because they are Mothers. "Woman is the mother of the race," gushed Boston feminist Julia Ward Howe, "the guardian of its helpless infancy, its earliest teacher, its most zealous champion. Woman is also the homemaker, upon her devolve the details which bless and beautify family life." And so on in paeans too painful to quote.

The women's movement dropped its earlier emphasis on opening up the profession to women: Why forsake Motherhood for the petty pursuits of males? And of course the impetus to attack professionalism itself as inherently sexist and elitist was long since dead. Instead, they turned to professionalizing women's natural functions. Housework was glamorized in the new discipline of "domestic science." Motherhood was held out as a vocation requiring much the same preparation and skill as nursing or teaching.

So while some women were professionalizing women's domestic roles, others were "domesticizing" professional roles, like nursing, teaching, and, later, social work. For the woman who chose to express her feminine drives outside of the home, these occupations were presented as simple extensions of women's "natural" domestic role. Conversely the woman who remained at home was encouraged to see herself as a kind of nurse, teacher, and counselor practicing within the limits of the family. And so the middle-class feminists of the late 1800s dissolved away some of the harsher contradictions of sexism.

THE DOCTOR NEEDS A NURSE

Of course, the women's movement was not in a position to decide on the future of nursing anyway. Only the medical profession was. At first, male doctors were a little skeptical about the new Nightingale nurses—perhaps suspecting that this was just one more feminine attempt to infiltrate medicine. But they were soon won over by the nurses' unflagging obedience. (Nightingale was a little obsessive on this point. When she arrived in the Crimea with her newly trained nurses, the doctors at first ignored them all. Nightingale refused to let her women lift a finger to help the thousands of sick and wounded soldiers until the doctors gave an order. Impressed, the doctors finally relented and set the nurses to cleaning up the hospital.) To the beleaguered doctors of the nineteenth century, nursing was a godsend: here at last was a kind of health worker who did not want to compete with the "regulars," did not have a medical doctrine to push, and who seemed to have no other mission in life but to serve.

While the average regular doctor was making nurses welcome, the new scientific practitioners of the early-twentieth century were making them *necessary*.

The new, post-Flexner physician was even less likely than his predecessors to stand around and watch the progress of his "cures." He diagnosed, he prescribed, he moved on. He could not waste his talents, or his expensive academic training in the tedious detail of bedside care. For this he needed a patient, obedient helper, someone who was not above the most menial tasks, in short a nurse.

Healing, in its fullest sense, consists of both curing and caring, doctoring *and* nursing. The old lay healers of an earlier time had combined both functions, and were valued for both. (For examples, midwives not only presided at the delivery, but lived in until the new mother was ready to resume care of her children.) But with the development of scientific medicine, and the modern medical profession, the two functions were split irrevocably. Curing became the exclusive province of the doctor; caring was relegated to the nurse. All credit for the patient's recovery went to the doctor and his "quick fix," for only the doctor participated in the mystique of Science. The nurse's activities, on the other hand, were barely distinguishable from those of a servant. She had no power, no magic, and no claim to the credit.

Doctoring and nursing arose as complementary functions, and the society which defined nursing as feminine could readily see doctoring as intrinsically "masculine." If the nurse was idealized Woman, the doctor was idealized Man—combining intellect and action, abstract theory, and hard-headed pragmatism. The very qualities which fitted Woman for nursing barred her from doctoring, and vice versa. Her tenderness and innate spirituality were out of place in the harsh, linear world of science. His decisiveness and curiosity made him unfit for long hours of patient nurturing.

These stereotypes have proved to be almost unbreakable. Today's leaders of the American Nursing Association may insist that nursing is no longer a feminine vocation but a neuter "profession." They may call for more male nurses to change the "image," insist that nursing requires almost as much academic preparation as medicine, and so on. But the drive to "professionalize" nursing is, at best, a flight from the reality of sexism in the health system. At worst, it is sexist itself, deepening the division among women health workers and bolstering a hierarchy controlled by men.

JOURNAL FOR NURSES

Happening
in Denver

upational Therapy

ase History
of a Dying Race

April 1956

Conclusion

WE HAVE OUR OWN MOMENT OF HISTORY TO WORK out, our own struggles. What can we learn from the past that will help us—in a Women's Health Movement—today?

These are some of our conclusions:

- We have not been passive bystanders in the history of medicine. The present system was born in and shaped by the competition between male and female healers. The medical profession in particular is not just another institution which happens to discriminate against us: it is a fortress designed and erected to exclude us. This means to us that the sexism of the health system is not incidental, not just the reflection of the sexism of society in general or the sexism of individual doctors. It is historically older than medical science itself; it is deep-rooted, institutional sexism.

- Our enemy is not just "men" or their individual male chauvinism: it is the whole class system which enabled male, upper-class healers to win out and which forced us into subservience. Institutional sexism is sustained by a class system which supports male power.

- There is no historically consistent justification for the exclusion of women from healing roles. Witches were attacked for being pragmatic, empirical, and immoral. But in the nineteenth century the rhetoric reversed: women became too unscientific, delicate, and sentimental. The *stereotypes* change to suit male convenience—*we* don't, and there is nothing in our "innate feminine nature" to justify our present subservience.

- Men maintain their power in the health system through their monopoly of scientific knowledge. We are mystified by science, taught to believe that it is hopelessly beyond our grasp. In our frustration, we are sometimes tempted to reject *science*, rather than to challenge the men who hoard it. But medical science could be a liberating force, giving us real control over our own bodies and power in our lives as health workers. At this point in our history, every effort to take hold of and share medical knowledge is a critical part of the struggle—know-your-body courses and literature, self-help projects, counseling, and women's free clinics.

- Professionalism in medicine is nothing more than the institutionalization of male upper-class monopoly. We must never confuse professionalism with expertise. Expertise is something to work for and to share; professionalism is—by definition—elitist and exclusive, sexist, racist, and classist. In the American past, women who sought formal medical training were too ready to accept the professionalism that went with it. They made *their* gains in status—but only on the backs of their less privileged sisters—midwives, nurses, and lay healers. Our goal today should never be to open up the exclusive medical profession to women, but to open up medicine—to all women.

- This means that we must begin to break down the distinctions and barriers between women health workers and women consumers. We should build shared concerns: consumers aware of women's needs as workers, workers in touch with women's needs as consumers. Women workers can play a leadership role in collective self-help and self-teaching projects, and in attacks on health institutions. But they need support and solidarity from a strong women's consumer movement.

- Our oppression as women health workers today is inextricably linked to our oppression as women. Nursing, our predominate role in the health system, is simply a workplace extension of our roles as wife and mother. The nurse is socialized to believe that rebellion violates not only her "professionalism," but her very femininity. This means that the male medical elite has a very special stake in the maintenance of sexism in the society at large: doctors are the bosses in an industry where the workers are primarily women. Sexism in the society at large insures that the female majority of the health workforce are "good" workers—docile and passive. Take away sexism and you take away one of the mainstays of the health hierarchy.

What this means to us in practice is that in the health system there is no way to separate worker organizing from feminist organizing. To reach out to women health workers *as workers* is to reach out to them as *women*.

Bibliography

[As appeared in the original 1973 printing.]

The Manufacture of Madness, by Thomas Szasz, MD, Delta Books, 1971. Szasz asserts that institutional psychiatry is the modern version of the witch-hunts, with the patient in the role of the witch. We are indebted to him for first presenting witchcraft in the context of the struggle between professionals and lay healers. See especially the chapter on "The Witch as Healer."

Satanism and Witchcraft, by Jules Michelet. The Citadel Press, 1939. A mid-nineteenth century work by a famous French historian. A vivid book on the Middle Ages, superstition and the Church, with a discussion of "satan as physician."

The Malleus Maleficarum, by Heinrich Kramer and James Sprenger, translated by Rev. Montague Summers. The Pushkin Press, London, 1928. Difficult medieval writing, but by far the best source for the day-to-day operations of the witch-hunts, and for insights into the mentality of the witch-hunter.

The History of Witchcraft and Demonology, by Rev. Montague Summers. University Books, New York, 1956. Written in the 1920s by a Catholic priest and defender—really!—of the witch-hunts. Attacks the witch as "heretic," "anarchist," and "bawd."

Witchcraft, by Pennethrone Hughes. Penguin Books, 1952. A general introduction and survey.

Women Healers in Medieval Life and Literature, by Muriel Joy Hughes. Books for Libraries Press,

Freeport, New York, 1943. A conservatively written book, with good information on the state of academic medicine and on women lay doctors and midwives. Unfortunately, it dismisses the whole question of witchcraft.

The Witch Cult in Western Europe, by Margaret Alice Murray. Oxford University Press, 1921. Dr. Murray was the first person to present the anthropological view, now widely accepted, that witchcraft represented, in part, the survival among the people of a pre-Christian religion.

A Mirror of Witchcraft, by Christina Hole. Catto and Windus, London, 1957. A source-book of extracts from trial reports and other writings, mostly from English witch trials of the sixteenth and seventeenth centuries.

The Formation of the American Medical Profession: The Role of Institutions, 1780-1860, by Joseph Kett. Yale University Press, 1968. Conservative point of view, but full of scattered information on lay healers. He discusses the politically radical nature of the Popular Health Movement in Chapter Four.

Medicine in America: Historical Essays, by Richard H. Shryock. Johns Hopkins Press, 1966. A readable, wide-ranging and fairly liberal book. See especially the chapters on "Women in American Medicine" and "The Popular Health Movement."

American Medicine and the Public Interest, by Rosemary Stevens. Yale University Press 1971. Long and dry, but useful for the early chapters on the formation of the American medical profession and the role of the foundations.

Medical Education in the US and Canada, by Abraham Flexner, Carnegie Foundation, 1910. (Available from University Microfilms, Ltd., Ann Arbor.) The famous "Flexner Report" that changed the face of American medical education. Some reasonable proposals, but amazing elitism, racism, and sexism.

The History of Nursing, by RIchard Shryock. N.B. Saunders, 1959. Better than most nursing histories—which are usually glorifications of nursing by nursing educators—but must worse than Shryock's medical histories.

Lonely Crusader: The Life of Florence Nightingale, by Cecil Woodham-Smith. McGraw Hill, 1951. A richly detailed biography which puts nursing in the context of the oppression of upper-class Victorian women.

Glances and Glimpses, by Harriet K. Hunt. Source Book Press, 1970. Rambling autobiography of a feminist and "irregular" woman doctor of the mid-nineteenth century. It's useful for its descriptions of the state of medical practice at the time.

"The American Midwife Controversy: A Crisis of Professionalization," by Frances E. Kobrin. *Bulletin of the History of Medicine,* July-August 1966, p.350. Restrained and scholarly account of the outlawing of American midwives. Very worthwhile reading.